Contents

Introduction
Is it hard to quit vaping?

Is vaping bad for your health? That's a difficult question; there is not yet a clear answer to whether or not vaping is bad for you, or whether it is actually healthier than smoking. However, vaping is addictive and will mostly turn into an addiction. Any addiction is a bad one, an addiction is feeling as if you need something to survive, which you don't actually need at all. You've lost some control over yourself, because your body has created a new need. Chapter 2 will elaborate some more on this subject.

Whether or not it is hard to quit vaping is something that depends on how you decide to try and quit. Stopping with vaping is not too hard, finding a method with which to successfully quit is. Your own motivation to stop vaping might be incredibly strong at the start of your effort to never touch an e-cigarette ever again. But will this internal motivation last for even a few weeks? Most of the time it will not, which is why a guide such as this would be the tool you need to stop vaping forever. I have stopped vaping with exactly the method this book will describe. Spoiler alert: I did not go to any doctor, I did not use any form of nicotine gum or patches, I did not even use any sort of product at all.

I used to vape each and every day, more than I would like to admit, for years on end. But now I don't vape at all. How did I do that? That's a question many people ask me when I tell them that I quit vaping. Well, I'm about to answer that question throughout this book and hope that your story will be nearly identical to mine after you have quit this addictive habit.

In this book I will show you how to quit Vaping in just 7 steps, some of which are surprisingly easy. But before that, I will speak a little about my thoughts on e-cigarettes, and what you might expect will happen to you when you quit vaping. But first will I dedicate some paragraphs to willpower. After having gone through these few subjects, I will show you step by step how I stopped vaping and how you will too.

I would wish you good luck on your journey, but I don't think you'll even need it.

Chapter 1
Willpower and rationality

Willpower plays a big role in your road to success and my method. However, it is not only a consistent medium to strong will you need to succeed; you also need to be rational. In all honesty, how much do you really enjoy vaping? And how often do you not enjoy vaping at all, but do so anyway? I guess that this is quite often, and if not you'll likely feel at least some form of guilt towards yourself after you have vaped, guilt that might feel like a lot of weight for you to carry on your shoulders. Do you really like being a vaper? Or are you addicted to it? You need to keep in mind what it is you are trying to stop with; not a joyous activity but rather a terrible habit.

You need not only to keep clear what you are going to remove from your life, but also what it is that you want. What is your goal? What is the outcome that you desire? If you keep this goal as clear as possible, you will succeed more easily than otherwise. Is your final goal to stop vaping? Yes. But what you want does not end there; you also want to be healthy, more energized, free of addiction, remove this heavy weight of guilt off of your shoulders, and feel strong for defeating this addiction. But most of all, the one thing everybody wants is progress. Progress is what makes happy, just doing anything at all that serves to progress yourself will make you feel better. Progress equals growth, and growth makes us feel alive. Progress towards this goal that you must see clearly. For step one you will make a list of motivations as to why you want to be vape-free, be sure to also write down on that list what your actual goals are.

When you start this process, you will notice how many people actually vape. You have probably experienced something like this before: how often have you bought a product and later saw how many people actually own that same product, whether headphones, clothing, or a car. You become more aware of what you do, or did in this case, and how many others do it as well. This awareness is caused by you trying to stop vaping and this awareness can make it quite difficult for you to keep going. It could very well be that you slip up one time or another. Having a slip and vaping for a bit is something you want to absolutely avoid. But, if you happen to slip up you are not automatically a vaper again. You should not return to vaping like you do right now just because you slipped up this one time. If you slip up, you must stand up again. Keep trying until you succeed. Keep trying and never give up. A baby will fall hundreds of times before he can actually walk. We don't tell a baby to stay down because it can't walk, we want him to keep trying until he eventually succeeds. Everybody has gone through this process, everyone in the world has. Whether when learning how to walk, write, tie shoelaces, or dress themselves; everyone has gone through this again and again. You have already succeeded in learning something, or doing something, that might have one day seemed impossible to you.

There is one thing many people fear when starting this journey to a vape-free lifestyle, and that would be to go through withdrawal. Vaping is like any other addiction; you think that e-cigarettes make you feel better. When you feel bad, vaping for a bit might cheer you up, you will feel a little better. When you have vaped a bit you might think "this vaping is what makes me feel better", but what most never think is "this vaping is what made me feel bad in the first place". Stopping doesn't make you feel bad, you have to put the blame on e-cigarettes. It is the e-cigarettes that make you feel bad when you stay away from them. The withdrawal symptoms might be harsh, and that is why you have to make sure you only experience them once. They are, after all, temporary symptoms. If you think you will fail this, you will fail. But, if you know you will succeed, you will succeed. You have to decide to stop, not just talk about it or keep pushing it to another date, you have to decide that you no longer want to vape.

My brother was reading a book some months ago which was titled "the four hour workweek". After he read it, I saw this book lying around and asked my brother what it was according to the writer you needed to do to achieve a four hour workweek, and still get wealthy. My brother said that to achieve such a four hour workweek, you will need to work almost every waking hour for a couple of years so as to get enough money and experience you can use to make any wealth increasing activity an automated process. And so it is with quitting vaping; you need to refuse to vape completely, until you automatically, and without thought, no longer desire to vape in the first place.

Chapter 2
Vaping is addictive

Before I started vaping c cigarettes, I would smoke Hookah. A Hookah is just a smoking "device" for which you do not use any drugs, a misconception I have to argue against almost any time I mention the use of a hookah. Yes, you can put weed in a hookah, as you can in a cigarette. But this is hardly important right now, what is important is that after I smoked Hookah, I turned to cigarettes, and after I had smoked cigarettes for years on end, I went to an electric-cigarette (also referred to often as a vaper).

It is not yet known how bad for your health the use of a vaper actually is. I've heard people stating that it is a terrible device for your health, and I've heard people stating that it's not that bad for you. However, it is not how bad it is for you that I want to discuss here. Rather, I want you to know that vaping is a terrible setback when you try to become free of addiction. Why would I make such a heavy statement? Because I know the following is true: A cigarette ends, it only takes about 5 minutes to smoke a cigarette after which you face the following decision: "Do I light another cigarette, or don't I?" This is what I would call a "natural stopping point" a point in the process of smoking when it feels most natural to stop smoking cigarettes for the time being, and go back inside or do something else. A vaper does not have this natural stopping point! There is not a time when you have finished your vaper apart from when the liquid needs to be replenished or your battery re-charged, and both of these might only occur every 6 hours. That's a stopping point every 360 minutes, while the stopping point for cigarettes is every 5 minutes and that of a hookah is once every 45 minutes.

You might think that I am exaggerating right now, but I am not. Your vape does not leave such a strong smell as your cigarette would do, so you can vape it inside your own home without bothering others, and many places allow you to vape while disallowing you to smoke. So why would you every stop? I did this myself as well, I sat behind my computer at home and took a drag every now and then (most often while waiting for an application to load or while watching some video's).

Vaping used to be the last thing I did before I closed my eyes, and the first thing I did every morning, this is no exaggeration. It is incredibly difficult to put away your vaper for even an hour or so, let alone for forever from now on. This is why I state that regardless of whether vaping might be worse, or less worse, for your health when compared to cigarettes or hookah's, they are absolutely worse for your route to being addiction free. Yes, a vaper is indeed addicting but I expect you know this because you are reading this book after all. Any addiction is unhealthy. If you are addicted to something, you can't life without what you are addicted to. Sure, there are people that say you are also addicted to air, because you need to breathe. Yes, that is true, but if you stop breathing you will die, and if you stop vaping you don't. That's the difference between being addicted and being required to perform certain actions to stay alive and healthy.

The same goes to being addicted to gambling, it sure isn't unhealthy for you physically but still very unhealthy for your mental stability and finances. Being addicted to shopping, or working, or sugar, are all undesirable. Whether they are mentally or physically unhealthy, they are bad for you; every addiction is bad for you because you lose a bit of self-control (or a lot). Indeed, beating an addiction is a fight to gain back some lost control over yourself.

Chapter 3

Effects of quitting

Vaping is seen as socially less acceptable now than it used to be; some employers prefer people who don't need to go on a vape break every hour or more, and many places do not allow you to vape inside anymore. It can also be more difficult to rent a home if you are a vaper and friends will likely ask you to not vape in their car or home. However, this is all avoidable if you quit vaping; you don't feel the need to Vape in someone's car, so you'll neither feel rejected when you're told you can't. The same goes for standing with other parents in front of a school, awaiting their children to get of school; some schools do not allow you to vape on the school area and you will therefore not be able to socialize with the parents of other children. The same goes for the sidelines of sport fields such as football or tennis, where you are no longer allowed to vape or other people will think of you less if you do. Also, if you are at a party or get-together at someone's place, and you want to vape but can't inside, you are required to go outside and step away from the festivities and interactions. You must socially isolate yourself in order to vape.

As a side note: not being a "vaper" will also make you more attractive to any possible love-interest, who might often see vaping as an instant turn-off.

Vaping can also have other negative effects on your credibility in numerous ways. If you vape while being a doctor, people will find this quite ironic and will likely think of it as hypocritical. The same goes for how strong people will think you are. Non-vapers will likely think of you as less strong because you are addicted to e-cigarettes. They might view you as unable to put your mind to something like quitting. And quitting an addiction might be more difficult than a non-Vaper thinks. Regardless, they might still think less of you in terms of how strong your will is. Also, if you tell people that you have quit vaping, many respect you all the more and will think of you as very strong-willed and a very responsible person.

Chapter 4
Step 1: Motivations

And now my guide begins in earnest. And guess what, you've already been busy with the first step of my guide since the very start of this book. The first thing you are required to do as per my method is creating a list of reasons why you want to stop vaping. Well, the actual first step would be that you'd have to admit to having an addiction and wanting to receive help for it, but since you've bought this book I presume you have already taken this step. The list you are going to create should be physical, digital, or preferably both, but not only mental.

This list you are going to create should consist of as many reasons as possible for you to stop vaping. Reasons already stated in this book can absolutely be used in your own list of reasons, if they are your reasons as well. The reason this list should be either physical or digital is because in a time of weakness, or great craving, you can definitively use such a list as a crutch to lean on. If this list is mental, you can and will forget certain motivations, something that will be impossible once they are present on a piece of paper. If you want to have such a list on a digital format, I suggest you use your phone to do so because of it being quite portable and probably on you at all times. The reasons for you to stop vaping could be of any kind: Biological, social, financial, spiritual, etc. But it would not be enough for such a list to consist only of "if you vape this happens" motivations; you'll also need to use "if you don't vape, these positive things will happen" kind of motivations, such as have been given earlier in this book as well (showing your strength and gaining back self-control). Dig deep and don't hold back when it comes to coming up with any and all eligible reasons for you to never vape again. And give this list to a friend as well, who can remind you of these reasons when you need social support from them.

Also, do you actually enjoy each and every time you vape? Many don't, and I often hear stories of people only enjoying it perhaps only a few times a week or day, they don't enjoy it most of the time, the other times they vape are just habitual. This is a very big point to make regarding your motivation to stop vaping: All of these negative effects because of a habit you have, which you do not even enjoy.

If you have trouble coming up with enough reasons to put on your list, you can definitely ask someone close to you for help, or look up more reasons to quit vaping online. However, you must fully agree with each and every reason to stop vaping on that list. They may be motivations given to you by someone else, but as long as you really belief in them being a reason to stop, it will work. If you write down reasons you don't really believe in, you'll only lengthen your list while making it a less compact or efficient document.

If you have a certain place somewhere where you usually vape, say the yard, balcony or a certain room, be certain to hang this list there as well (if it is a private place), so that it may serve as the last stand of defense in your effort, you will be stopped by this list. The entire process of quitting starts with, and relies upon, your motivation and your wish to go through with this process until you no longer desire any sort of vaping. You absolutely can do this! You just need to want it enough, and with such a list you'll keep reminding yourself that this is definitely what you want. The only one that can decide whether to go through with this, or give in, is you. Believe in yourself, you can do it, I could too and I am by no means extraordinary.

Chapter 5
Step 2: Support

The social support you can get from others has been very briefly mentioned in the previous chapter when there was being spoken of getting help thinking of reasons not to vape anymore. However, that is not the only effect social support can have on this process. I encourage you to find out who in your direct surroundings can, and are willing to, support you in your cause. If you promise these people that you will stop vaping, you'll have a promise to live up to not just made to yourself, but to others as well.

Also, whenever you feel the need to vape again, you can ask these people to help you refrain from doing so. These people can tell you why you shouldn't vape according to yourself, not just according to them and other people. To reach this effect I suggest you share the list you created during the first step of this process. If you let people around you know that you want to quit vaping, why not go a small step further and ask them to help you by not vaping around you too much? Or at the very least, tell them not to ask you if you to go vaping. It is already difficult enough to say no to your own mind when it asks you whether to vape or not, let alone when other people ask you as well.

Furthermore, if you are somewhere other than at your own home, you should not carry any e-cigarettes or with you so that, if you want to vape, you don't have anything on you with which to do so. If you have told your friends about your goals of not vaping anymore you can ask them all you'd like whether you can borrow their e-cigarette or not, but if they are reasonable and loyal they won't give you any. By letting people around you know what you are going through, they'll also take it as less offensive when you get annoyed more often and more quickly around them, or get more stressed and anxious, because they'll know what is going on. You can also let them know that, as has been shown earlier in this book, you'll likely only act like this for 2 to 4 weeks, a relatively short time.

The very best effect social support might have would be other people willing to join you on your journey; perhaps this was just that little push in the right direction they needed to stop vaping themselves as well. This process will get a lot easier when you'll go through it with someone else who has the same goal. You can inspire each other and will be less willing to fail, because you would not only disappoint yourself, and those others you have told about this, but you will also leave your companions behind to face their troubles on their own. However a companion might be a catalyst for you to carry on your fight, they can also be a catalyst for you to give up. When both companions speak of wanting to give up, they might end up convincing the other and themselves to quit this process. This is a trap you must not fall for! If the other so desperately wants to fail, and you have tried all you could to prevent this from happening, then you should let them fail on their own and not fail with them.

Chapter 6
Step 3: Choose a start

Choosing a date to start this process is more important, and takes more thought, than you might initially assume. Having a starting date will mean that you have only a limited amount of time to prepare yourself. This might sound like a bad thing, but in reality, it is not. Because of your limited amount of time you will start to work on those preparations sooner rather than later, you can't push it off too much. If you don't have a starting date, you'll just push of that date until you are prepared. You will take preparing slow, and easy. By having a starting date, you will start preparing as soon as possible so that, when your journey finally starts, you still have all the things you did to prepare yourself freshly present within your mind. If you were to create the list from step one today, and only start this journey in 3 months, you will have forgotten why certain reasons on that list are important to you, because you did not start using it soon enough after you wrote it. You should not rush yourself mind you, rushing might decrease the quality of your preparation, but you should stay focused on your goal.

Be careful about choosing a date, make sure that the date you choose is not also a date when you'll go to a festival, a music performance, or any other place where there are a lot of people vaping. There is no need to make your first day off the e-cigarettes one of the hardest. However, you can also view such a day as a gigantic challenge, and if you manage to not vape on such a day you can feel certain that you can beat any day ahead of you as well.

The preparations for this journey can all be done within a few days, so if you are ready to quit vaping sooner than expected, by all means go for it. Furthermore, make sure that the date you stop vaping is a special day; remember the date, do something to celebrate your start of this journey, make it a day to enjoy but also a day which you do not want to spoil by vaping later on anyway. Often, the most difficult part of reaching a goal is the starting of the process that is needed to succeed. This is true for what you are about to do, but also goes for sporting, writing a book, starting to study, starting with painting, etc., etc. If you put your date to far ahead, you might start to dread it as the day comes nearer, the earlier you get over this invisible barrier, the better.

Chapter 7
Step 4: Invest

Investments always consist of resources, energy, or time. If you make an investment, you want these resources to have exceeded their initial value by the end of any project you have invested in. and so it is with vaping. And therefore the day you quit should be an investment. By making it an investment you'll lose more if you give in and vape again, which is why you'll need to make a bigger investment so you'll never go back to vaping again because, if you do, it'll cost you a lot of resources. You need to throw away all that you own and is used to vape. If you want to start vaping again, you'll need to repurchase all these items again, which will make you more hesitant to go through with it at all. This helped me the most when I stopped vaping, I simply destroyed my vaper. The investment of a broken vaper made me reluctant to start again because I would need to pay around twenty bucks if I'd do so. So, I didn't start vaping again.

Apart from throwing stuff away being an investment, you can also view it as removing reminders and items that awaken cravings in you. If you see any e-liquids, you'll be reminded of e-cigarettes and might want to start vaping again. It is hard enough as it is to fight these cravings and reminders when you walk outside and see people vaping, or see people vaping on television or the internet. By throwing these things away, you'll at least do away with the nearest tempting items. Doing away with all of these vape-related items might be something you want to, more or less, ceremoniously do on the day you vape for the last time, this is totally fine but please do collect the items you want to discard beforehand.

If you have someone living with you who vapes, ask them if they would put their own items in an unreachable or unseen place so as to aid you. These could be places like saves, locked drawers, or under their bed.

Finally, do not save one bottle of liquid and a e-cigarette "just in case you really need to vape", without those items in your possession this "case" might never even become a reality, and if it does you'll beat it or lose your investments.

Chapter 8
Step 5: Avoid

As soon as you stop vaping, you will notice how many people around you vape. These people could be close friends, colleagues, or anyone at all for that matter. It is a classic case of not noticing something until you don't have it anymore. Especially when it is turning spring or summer, a lot of people will be sitting outside and vaping on terraces, beaches, or wherever. But also when it's not summer, when you're just walking outside you'll see people vaping, when you're driving your car you'll see other drivers vape, when you'll watch TV you'll see people vaping, this all makes it incredibly hard to not think about it. It might be best to avoid these places of frequent vaping if possible, at least when you get cravings or at the start of your journey to a vape-free life.

Yes, seeing other people vaping can be a trigger for your cravings to start growing. But whenever you'll walk among them, remind yourself of why it is you don't vape, why it is that you don't want to let your life be ruled by those small sticks on which they suck, be proud of yourself for not vaping and kindly refusing to do so if anyone were to off you a vape. When people come to your place, don't let them vape there, especially after having made those investments mentioned earlier. If you get caught in a place with vapers and find yourself wanting to vape anyway, go outside or to another room until the urge passes.

Avoid going on a vape-break, rather take a coffee or tea brake instead so that you still consume something, taste something, and have something to do with your hands. This way you'll also meet other people who also go on a break of another kind than that of a vape-break.

However, seeing other people vape is not the only trigger you will experience. Being bored is another major contributor to your wish to be vaping. A personal example of mine would be when I would wait on a train, or the bus. How do you pass the time waiting on a bus or something? You'll vape, solely because you are bored at that moment. But, there are other things you can do while waiting such as reading a book, texting people, fill in a crossword puzzle or Sudoku, play a game on your phone, call someone, walk around a bit and go to some stores if you have to wait for longer periods of time, go write something down such as a grocery list or to-do list, or go look at some videos on your phone. Most of the things I have just mentioned only require a mobile phone, just download some puzzles or a book, or go on the internet and watch some clips, you really don't need to carry a (puzzle)book with you. Lately I have been playing Mastermind on my phone when I'm bored and not at home, it's as simple as that. But if you don't fill this time you normally used to vape with another activity, it will get very hard on you indeed.

The consumption of alcohol will enlarge certain cravings you have, and weaken your ability to resist them. This also goes for the craving of having a e-cigarette. If you want to succeed at quitting, you'll do better to avoid drinking for the first few weeks of this process. In your preparation stage, try to go out drinking the same as you might normally do, but without vaping. This way you'll be prepared a bit more for when you actually stop.

Other times in your day you might usually Vape could be after meals. If so, after a meal go brush your teeth right away so you'll not only ruin your breath if you do have vape, but also so that you'll change your routine a bit. The same goes for when you drink coffee; many vapers drink coffee and vape at the same time, try to do something else while drinking coffee such as solving a puzzle, or for the very brave: go brush your teeth as well. Keep your mind away from e-cigarettes and on something else, as should you do regarding your hands. The same goes for when you're watching a movie, or are behind your computer, instead of vaping, suck on a lollipop, take a mint, or cough drop. You'll feel the desire to vape fade away.

Chapter 9
Step 6: Milestones

Now that you have stopped vaping, even if just for a single day, you can be proud of yourself. Even just having not vaped for 24 hours might just be the longest period of no-vaping you've had in years, let alone not vaping for 4 days. Be proud of yourself, and celebrate the strength you obviously have because you have the power to stop vaping. Every day should be celebrated, but you should also set some milestones such as not having vaped anything for a week, month, three months, year, etc. Do not make your next milestone too distant; it will seem to be unreachable. If you buy yourself something as a reward for not Vaping, you should display it somewhere as if it is a trophy, because you have earned it as if it were a trophy. If you feel guilty about spoiling yourself, don't! Rewards should be over the top and you have earned it all by yourself. If you have stopped vaping together with someone else, you can also decide to buy each other a gift, or treat each other in another way, after having reached certain milestones. Giving yourself a reward that will further boost your confidence are of the best kind, since they will give you more strength to keep away from the e-cigarettes. Confidence boosts like these could be some cool outfits, get a new haircut, or take some classes you've always wanted.

You can also reward yourself for living a vape-free live by going to concerts (keep the tickets as trophy), buy equipment for a hobby (such as a new fishing rod, or a new camera), buy a plant every week you haven't vaped, try a new restaurant or go to a familiar one, see a movie, buy some expensive food and enjoy cooking it, go on a road trip, buy a new game, or throw a party.

The most important gift you get from not Vaping is that you have proven to yourself that you are resilient, motivated, brave, strong, hardworking, determined, courageous, independent and unstoppable.

Chapter 10
Step 7: Never vape again

The final step you have to take is to never vape again, it sounds difficult yes, but when you've managed to not vape for a month, or perhaps a few, you can manage to never vape again as well. There will be times when it will get though, but even then it will never get as hard as the first few days again.

Make sure all of your investments have been worth it, including the investment of having been through the withdrawal symptoms. And when you feel like giving up, just remember to check the list you have made as described as the very first step of this process. Or let those you have chosen to support you remind you of this list. If that doesn't help either, at least you have invested too much to lose just because your body thinks it needs to vape. If you give up, you will not only fail to deliver on your promise to your friends and yourself, you will also nullify all your investments and efforts, you'll have thrown away all that you had related to vaping just to need to buy it again now, and you will lose the rewards you have promised yourself at the milestones. But above all, you will lose your self-respect or at least the respect for yourself you could have had, had you gone through with it. But there is no way you will lose all of this, because you will not give up.

Chapter 11
After you have stopped

When you vape, you are a vaper; it is a part of your personality at that time, a bad part. The more you vape the bigger the part it plays. If you stop vaping, you change a part of your personality for the better. I shall now mention some of these changes.

First of all, you will no longer understand why you used to vape as much as you did. vaping will no longer seem attractive to you, especially after you have realized you could stop doing so. You will also stop thinking about vaping at all, it will no longer play a part in your life at all, not even in the back of your mind for most of the time. But when you do think about vaping, you will feel sick. You will feel sick when thinking about vaping and how it would feel like it would clog your throat if you did.

Another side effect of having stopped vaping might be that you experience some nightmares in which you vape, and have failed to stop, after all what you have done. I am not the only one who has experienced these nightmares, many people who I spoke to about these dreams have told me that they have dreamt the same dreams. Luckily, it is a nightmare you wake up from.

A thank you

I would like to end this book by thanking all of those who have supported me while writing this book, as well as my other books.

But even more so do I want to thank everybody who has helped me to quit vaping. Although harsh, your guidance has led me to where I am now, and for that I am thankful.

Books by this author

Be sure to join the mail group by emailing
theimprovinglifeproject@hotmail.com to receive
updates, ask questions, and more! Please leave a
message, or a review on Amazon.

Books by this Jim Sonofsil:

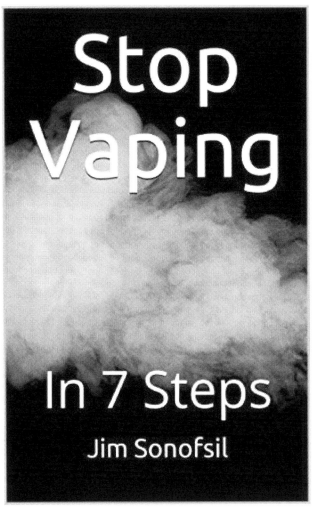

Stop Vaping: In 7 Steps
$ 3.45 Kindle
$ 7.50 Paperback
https://www.amazon.com/dp/B07G9NPP4Hv

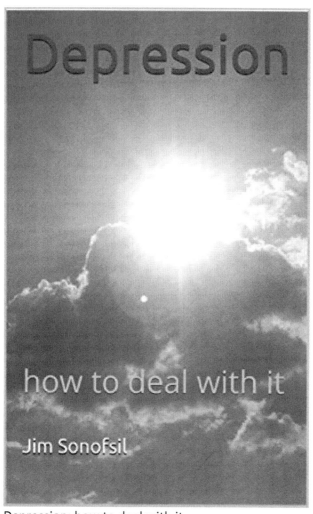

Depression: how to deal with it
$ 3.42 Kindle
$9.50 Paperback
https://www.amazon.com/dp/B07DK7629S

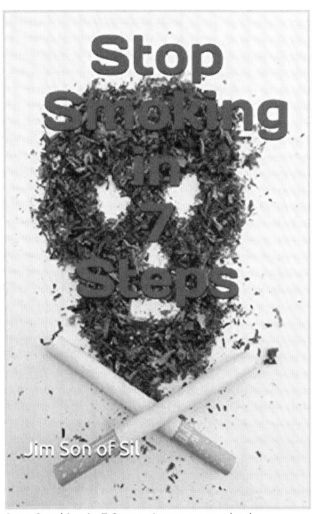

Stop Smoking in 7 Steps: A proven method
$ 3.48 Kindle
$ 10.00 Paperback
https://www.amazon.com/dp/B07F191XHH

Life Hack
$ 3.46 Kindle
$ 5.55 Paperback
https://www.amazon.com/dp/B07G6MD1RC

Your Child's Potential: Math Age 3 to 8
$ 3.48 Kindle
$ 7.50 Paperback
https://www.amazon.com/dp/1718127782

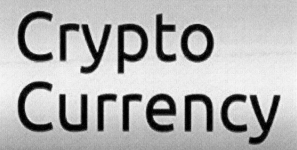

Crypto currency: How to invest in Bitcoin, Ethereum, Dash, and many more
$3.42 Kindle
$7.50 paperback
https://www.amazon.com/dp/B07GNWDP2J

Printed in Great Britain
by Amazon

73342899R00024